SCIATICA SOLUTIONS

Therapies for Nerve Pain Relief and Spinal Health

Find Relief From Sciatica With Therapeutic Solutions Targeting Nerve Pain And Promoting Overall Spinal Health

JAMES JOSEPH

Table of Contents

CHAPTER ONE

Introduction

Many people suffer from sciatica, which causes pain, stiffness, and a variety of symptoms that may have a substantial influence on their everyday lives.

Understanding the underlying causes, symptoms, medical diagnosis, and possible therapies is critical for individuals struggling with or hoping to avoid sciatica. This detailed examination delves into the complexities of sciatica, including its origins, symptoms, medical diagnosis, orthodox treatments, and alternative therapies such as physical therapy and chiropractic care.

Understanding Sciatica: Causes And Symptoms.

Sciatica is a phrase used to describe pain that spreads down the length of the sciatic nerve, the longest nerve in the body. The sciatic nerve runs from the lower back to the hips, buttocks, and down both legs. The most frequent cause of sciatica is compression or inflammation of the sciatic nerve, which is typically caused by a variety of underlying disorders.

Common causes of sciatic nerve compression include herniated discs, spinal stenosis, and bone spurs. A herniated disc occurs when the soft inner core of a spinal disc leaks out, irritating nearby nerves such as the sciatica.

Spinal stenosis is the narrowing of the spinal canal, while bone spurs are bony growths that may form on the vertebrae and possibly impinge on the sciatic nerve.

Sciatica symptoms are unique, and characterized by pain, tingling, or numbness that extends from the lower back down the buttocks and leg. The discomfort may range from moderate to severe, and it may intensify with extended sitting, standing, or movement.

Medical Diagnosis Of Sciatica: What To Expect

Sciatica is diagnosed after a comprehensive evaluation by

a healthcare expert, which frequently begins with a complete medical history to determine the start and type of the symptoms. A physical examination may involve evaluating muscular strength, reflexes, and range of motion. X-rays, MRIs, or CT scans may be ordered to confirm the diagnosis and determine the underlying reason.

These diagnostic technologies let doctors see the spine and identify problems including herniated discs, spinal stenosis, and other structural abnormalities that might be damaging the sciatic nerve. A correct diagnosis is essential for devising an effective treatment plan specific to the individual's condition.

CHAPTER TWO

Traditional Treatments For Sciatica: Pros And Cons

The typical approach to sciatica management often includes a mix of medicine, physical therapy, and, in rare situations, surgical intervention. Nonsteroidal anti-inflammatory medications (NSAIDs), such as ibuprofen or naproxen, may be used to treat pain and inflammation. muscular relaxants may also assist in relieving sciatica-related muscular spasms.

In more severe situations, corticosteroid injections directly into the afflicted region may be advised to decrease inflammation and offer temporary comfort. While drugs might give symptomatic relief, they may not treat the underlying cause of sciatica, and long-term usage can be linked with negative effects.

In situations when conservative therapy does not

give significant relief, surgical alternatives may be explored. Procedures such as discectomy (removing part of a herniated disc) or laminectomy (removing a portion of the spinal bone to reduce pressure) try to address the structural abnormalities causing sciatic nerve compression.

However, surgery is usually reserved for cases in which other therapies have failed and the benefits exceed the dangers.

Physical Therapy And Exercise For Sciatica Relief

Physical therapy is essential for controlling sciatica because it focuses on strengthening the muscles that support the spine, increasing flexibility, and resolving postural difficulties. A trained physical therapist can create a specific workout plan to relieve sciatic pain and avoid repeat occurrences.

Stretches to increase lower back and leg flexibility, as

well as strengthening exercises for the core and lower back muscles, are popular sciatica therapy activities. In addition, posture correction and body mechanics instruction are essential components of physical therapy for reducing spinal strain and promoting proper alignment.

Regular exercise, even low-impact sports like walking or swimming, may improve general spinal health and aid with weight management, which is critical for lowering strain on the sciatic nerve. While physical therapy has many advantages, consistency, and attention to the recommended exercises are essential for long-term recovery.

Chiropractic Care: Spinal Alignment For Nerve Pain Relief

Chiropractic therapy is an alternative technique that focuses on the musculoskeletal system, namely the spine, to relieve pain and improve general health. Chiropractors think that spinal misalignments, known as subluxations, may interfere with the nervous system's correct functioning, resulting in pain and other health disorders.

Chiropractic adjustments, also known as spinal manipulations, entail applying controlled force to particular joints in the spine to restore appropriate alignment. Chiropractors often treat sciatica by focusing on the lumbar spine to relieve pressure on the sciatic nerve and related symptoms.

Chiropractic therapy for sciatica aims to enhance spinal mobility and promote healthy nerve function. Chiropractors provide adjustments that are specific to the individual's condition and are often followed with lifestyle and ergonomic recommendations to avoid future problems.

While some people experience great comfort with chiropractic therapy, it is important to recognize that the efficacy of this technique varies. Chiropractic adjustments are typically regarded as safe when administered by a skilled and certified practitioner. Individuals with certain health concerns or who are uncomfortable with manual adjustments may choose other chiropractic treatments, such as instrument-assisted adjustments.

In conclusion, sciatica is a common and frequently severe ailment that may have a substantial influence on a person's quality of life. Understanding the origins, symptoms, and possible therapies is critical to properly treating and avoiding sciatic pain. While standard therapies like medication and surgery have their uses, alternative techniques like physical therapy and chiropractic care provide non-invasive solutions for pain relief and general spinal health. As with any medical problem, people should speak with healthcare specialists to identify the best treatment approach for their situation.

Yoga And Sciatica: Gentle Exercises For Spine Health

Yoga, an ancient discipline that harmonizes the body and mind, is now recognized for its therapeutic effects in the treatment of sciatica. Yoga is an excellent choice for those who want to relieve sciatic nerve pain since it emphasizes gentle movements, stretching, and regulated breathing.

Yoga positions for the lower back and hips may help relieve sciatica pain. Child's Pose, Cat-Cow Stretch, and Pigeon Pose are believed to increase spine flexibility and relieve stress in the afflicted regions. A regular yoga program not only increases flexibility but also strengthens the core muscles, which provide superior spinal support.

Mindfulness and meditation as part of yoga may help with stress reduction, which is important in controlling sciatica. Stress often exacerbates pain, and applying relaxation methods may result in a decrease in both physical and mental strain.

While yoga provides a mild and comprehensive approach to sciatica treatment, it is critical to speak with a healthcare expert or a trained yoga teacher before beginning a yoga practice, particularly if the practitioner is new to the discipline or has pre-existing health concerns.

CHAPTER THREE

Acupuncture And Alternative Treatments For Sciatica

Acupuncture, based on ancient Chinese medicine, involves putting tiny needles into certain sites on the body to increase energy flow or "qi." In the case of sciatica, acupuncture seeks to relieve pain and promote recovery.

According to research, acupuncture may help lower the severity and frequency of sciatica symptoms by altering the nerve system and producing endorphins, the body's natural analgesics.

Aside from acupuncture, alternative treatments such as chiropractic adjustments and massage therapy are gaining popularity for their potential advantages

in treating sciatica. Chiropractors adjust the spine to relieve pressure on the sciatic nerve, while massage treatment reduces muscular tension and promotes relaxation.

These alternative treatments, when combined with a thorough treatment plan, may provide relief and enhance overall well-being. Individual reactions vary, so it's important to speak with healthcare specialists to establish the best method for each person's specific requirements.

Medications For Sciatica Management: An Overview

Medications play an important role in sciatica management, attempting to relieve pain, decrease inflammation, and treat the underlying causes. Nonsteroidal anti-inflammatory medications (NSAIDs), such as ibuprofen and naproxen, are widely used to decrease inflammation and relieve pain.

However, long-term usage should be carefully managed to prevent any possible negative effects.

Oral corticosteroids may be administered to treat severe

pain by reducing inflammation surrounding the damaged nerve. muscular relaxants may help relieve the muscular spasms that typically accompany sciatica, resulting in increased comfort.

In certain circumstances, doctors may prescribe neuropathic drugs like gabapentin or pregabalin to treat nerve pain. These drugs function by regulating electrical activity in the nerves, relieving shooting and burning sensations.

Individuals must collaborate closely with healthcare specialists to select the best pharmaceutical regimen for them, taking into account aspects such as the intensity of their symptoms, general health, and possible drug interactions.

Sciatica-Friendly Diet And Lifestyle Changes

Dietary and lifestyle changes may have a major influence on sciatica treatment by improving general health and lowering inflammation. A well-balanced diet high in anti-inflammatory foods, such as fruits, vegetables, and fatty fish, may help to reduce pain and suffering.

Individuals with sciatica must maintain a healthy weight since excess weight puts strain on the spine and exacerbates nerve-related symptoms.

Hydration is another essential component of a sciatica-friendly lifestyle. Staying hydrated helps the spinal discs absorb trauma and preserve flexibility. Caffeine and alcohol use should be limited since they might cause dehydration and perhaps increase sciatic nerve discomfort.

Incorporating ergonomic measures into everyday living, such as keeping an appropriate posture and utilizing supportive furniture, may minimize lower back strain and help with long-term sciatica care.

CHAPTER FOUR

Heat And Cold Treatments For Sciatic Nerve Relief

Heat and cold treatments are simple but powerful ways to manage sciatic nerve pain, providing comfort via opposing effects on the body.

Heat treatment, which is often used using hot packs or warm baths, helps to relax muscles and enhance blood circulation. This may relieve muscular spasms and stiffness in the lower back and hips, making sciatica sufferers more comfortable.

Cold treatment, such as using ice packs or cold compresses, may help decrease inflammation and numb the afflicted region. Cold therapies are especially effective during acute episodes of sciatic nerve pain, providing a natural and drug-free alternative to control symptoms.

Individual tastes may differ, and some people find comfort in alternately using heat and cold therapy. To avoid damage, these treatments should be used with caution, for brief periods, and without direct contact with the skin.

Finally, sciatica treatment takes a comprehensive strategy that considers physical, emotional, and behavioral factors.

Individuals can experiment with a variety of strategies to find what works best for their specific needs, including the gentle movements of yoga, the ancient practice of acupuncture, medications prescribed by healthcare professionals, dietary changes, and the use of heat and cold therapies. Individuals who embrace a complete approach to sciatica therapy may recover control of their lives while also improving their spine health and general well-being.

Ergonomics And Posture: Preventing And Relieving Sciatic Pain

Sciatic pain, which causes discomfort along the sciatic nerve that travels down the lower back and into the legs, may have a substantial influence on a person's quality of life. While many variables contribute to sciatica, keeping proper ergonomics and posture is critical for avoiding and treating the illness.

Poor ergonomics and posture, whether at work or during

everyday activities, may put undue stress on the spine, resulting in sciatic discomfort. To solve this, people might use ergonomic principles to create a more supporting environment for their body.

Start by making sure your workstation is ergonomically sound. Adjust the height of your chair and workstation to produce a neutral spine posture while maintaining the spine's natural curvature. Use lumbar support to maintain your lower back's natural arch and avoid the possibility of sciatic nerve compression. Furthermore, taking frequent intervals to stand, stretch, and change postures might help to reduce stiffness and improve circulation, lowering the risk of sciatic discomfort.

When Is Surgical Treatment For Sciatica Necessary?

In circumstances when conservative therapy fails to produce relief, surgical surgery may be considered for sciatica management. Surgical methods seek to treat the underlying reasons for sciatic pain, which may include herniated discs, spinal stenosis, or other structural abnormalities.

Microdiscectomy is a frequent surgical treatment performed to treat sciatica caused by a herniated disc. In this minimally invasive procedure, a tiny part of the herniated disc is removed to relieve pressure on the sciatic nerve. Another possibility is spinal decompression surgery, which seeks to increase the space surrounding the damaged nerve roots.

While surgery may be useful in certain circumstances, it is usually reserved for cases when conservative methods have failed and the person is experiencing chronic and severe symptoms. Consulting with a healthcare practitioner is critical to determining if surgery is suitable depending on the patient's unique diagnosis and general condition.

Mind-Body Techniques For Dealing With Sciatic Nerve Pain

Beyond physical therapies, mind-body approaches may be quite helpful in controlling and living with sciatic nerve discomfort. Mindfulness meditation, deep breathing techniques, and guided visualization may help people shift their attention away from discomfort and relax.

Mindfulness meditation entails developing awareness of the current moment without judgment.

Individuals may separate from the severity of sciatic pain by concentrating their attention on breathing, sensations, or mental imagery. Similarly, deep breathing techniques may activate the body's relaxation response, lowering muscular tension and producing a sensation of peace.

Guided imagery is imagining relaxing sights or doing mental activities to divert the mind from pain. Individuals with sciatica who include these mind-body practices into their everyday routines might create coping strategies to deal with the problems of chronic pain and enhance their general well-being.

CHAPTER FIVE

Long-Term Strategies To Prevent Sciatica Recurrence

Preventing sciatica recurrence requires long-term measures that treat the underlying causes of the ailment. Regular exercise, especially exercises that strengthen core muscles and increase flexibility, is critical for maintaining spinal health and avoiding sciatic nerve compression.

Maintaining a healthy weight is another important part of avoiding sciatica recurrence.

Excess body weight may put more strain on the spine, worsening sciatic discomfort. Adopting a balanced and healthy diet, together with frequent physical exercise, may help with weight control and general spinal health.

Individuals with a history of sciatica should also be aware of their everyday routines and avoid actions that might worsen their disease.

This includes lifting heavy things with good form, avoiding extended sitting, and implementing ergonomic concepts into their regular routines.

Sciatica Treatments For Pregnant Women

Pregnancy typically causes changes in the body that might lead to sciatic discomfort. As the baby develops, the growing uterus may exert pressure on the sciatic nerve, causing discomfort and agony. However, some various tactics and remedies are particularly designed for pregnant women with sciatica.

Prenatal yoga and mild stretching activities may help relieve sciatic discomfort when pregnant. These exercises aim to increase flexibility, strengthen the core, and promote appropriate posture, all of which help to relieve strain on the sciatic nerve.

Pregnancy pillows and cushions may give support when sitting or sleeping, therefore promoting healthy spinal alignment. Furthermore, prenatal massage and physical therapy may help by reducing muscular tension and boosting relaxation.

Pregnant women with sciatica should talk with their healthcare practitioners before applying any new measures to ensure that the selected techniques are safe for both mother and baby.

Sciatica In Athletes: Specialised Approaches To Recovery

Athletes may be prone to sciatica as a result of repeated motions, muscular imbalances, or overuse injuries. Athletes may use specialized healing procedures to treat sciatic pain and prevent it from recurring, enabling them to continue competing at their peak.

Sports-specific training regimens that target core muscular strength, flexibility, and biomechanical asymmetries may help athletes avoid sciatica. Working with a sports medicine expert or physical therapist may assist in personalizing these regimens to an athlete's specific demands and requirements.

Targeted stretching practices, particularly for the muscles around the sciatic nerve, may help to increase flexibility and relieve pressure on the nerve. Furthermore, athletes should practice adequate warm-up and cool-down techniques before and after training or competition to reduce the risk of injury and sciatic discomfort.

In the event of sciatic pain, athletes should emphasize rest and recuperation, giving their bodies enough time to recuperate. This might include changing training regimens, integrating low-impact activities, and obtaining expert advice for recovery exercises.

To summarize, treating sciatic pain requires a diverse

strategy that includes ergonomic practices, mind-body approaches, surgical choices where needed, and customized solutions for certain populations such as pregnant women and sports. Individuals who take a complete approach to sciatica prevention and treatment may improve their overall health and have an active and satisfying life.

Living with sciatica may be a difficult journey, impacting not just physical but also mental health. This illness, which is distinguished by pain radiating down the sciatic nerve, needs meticulous therapy to offer a comprehensive approach to well-being. In this inquiry, we will look at the many facets of maintaining mental well-being while living with sciatica.

CHAPTER SIX
Managing Work and Daily Life with Sciatic Pain

Sciatica has a significant effect on everyday life, affecting many facets of one's routine in addition to physical pain. Managing sciatic pain while juggling professional commitments may be especially difficult for employees. Prolonged sitting, which is frequent in desk work, may increase sciatic discomfort.

Individuals suffering from sciatica may need to make

ergonomic alterations to their work environment to deal with this issue. Investing in an ergonomic chair, adjusting the desk height, and taking regular breaks for stretching and walking can all make a big difference.

Open communication with employers about the disease may develop understanding and, in some cases, lead to adjustments that improve the work environment for managing sciatic pain.

Aside from the job, everyday tasks such as transportation, domestic duties, and leisure hobbies may be affected. Developing a thoughtful attitude to movement, practicing good body mechanics, and requesting help when necessary may all contribute to a more sustainable daily routine.

Activities that enhance flexibility and strength, such as mild yoga or swimming, may help manage sciatica while also increasing general well-being.

Sciatica In Seniors: Personalized Approaches For Older Adults

Seniors with sciatic pain may encounter particular issues owing to age-related variables such as decreased bone density and joint flexibility.

It is critical to adjust management tactics to meet the special demands of older persons. Gentle exercises, mobility aids, and living space adaptations may all help seniors with sciatica improve their quality of life.

Seniors with sciatica must maintain a healthy lifestyle that includes a balanced diet and frequent exercise within their capabilities. Furthermore, mind-body techniques such as meditation or tai chi may benefit both physical and emotional well-being.

Regular contact with healthcare specialists ensures that treatment regimens are changed to reflect any age-related health concerns.

Sciatica In Children And Adolescents: Understanding Unique Challenges

While sciatica is generally linked with adults, children, and teenagers may also get the ailment, albeit less often. Understanding the particular issues that younger people with sciatica confront is critical to successful care.

Sciatica in children may be caused by congenital disorders, accidents, or anatomical abnormalities. Adolescents, on the other hand, may develop sciatica owing to development concerns or participation in particular activities. In these circumstances, diagnosis and therapy must be approached with caution, taking into account the growing musculoskeletal system.

Parents and caregivers have an important role in helping children and adolescents with sciatica. Creating a climate that promotes open discussion about pain and discomfort is critical. Seeking quick medical treatment, participating in age-appropriate physical activities, and making lifestyle changes are all important aspects of controlling sciatica in this cohort.

Sciatica And Mental Health: Connections And Coping Strategies

The complex relationship between sciatica and mental health cannot be ignored. Chronic pain typically causes emotional discomfort, such as irritation, worry, and even despair. The chronic nature of sciatic pain may disturb sleep, restrict movement, and make it difficult to participate in pleasant activities, all of which add to the emotional toll.

Coping skills for both the physical and emotional elements of sciatica are critical. Seeking help from mental health specialists, support groups, or counseling services may provide people with strategies to deal with the emotional effects of chronic pain. Mindfulness-based activities, such as meditation and deep breathing exercises, are effective tools for dealing with pain and maintaining mental health.

Participating in activities that offer pleasure and a feeling of success might serve as a counterweight to the difficulties presented by sciatica. Creative endeavors, hobbies, and quality time with loved ones all improve mental wellness. Individuals suffering from sciatica must understand the interdependence of their physical and mental well-being and actively explore treatments that address both.

Conclusion: Create A Comprehensive Sciatica Management Plan

Finally, maintaining emotional well-being with sciatica requires a holistic strategy that takes into account all elements of everyday living. A successful management plan includes navigating job duties, addressing the various obstacles experienced by elders and young people, and acknowledging the link between sciatica and mental health.

Building a support network that includes healthcare professionals, employers, family, and friends is critical for those suffering from sciatica. Individuals with sciatic pain may improve their overall well-being and live satisfying lives by adopting ergonomic improvements, age-appropriate therapies, and mental health techniques. Individuals may manage the complications of sciatica by taking a comprehensive and customized approach, which promotes not only physical resilience but also mental strength and vitality.